While every precaution has been taken in the preparation of this book, the publisher assumes no responsibility for errors or omissions, or for damages resulting from the use of the information contained herein.

IF THINGS COULD SING: A LOOK INTO HOSPICE MUSIC THERAPY

First edition. November 11, 2025.

Copyright © 2025 Miranda Wall MT-BC.

AF715305

ISBN: 979-8231118663

Written by Miranda Wall MT-BC.

If Things Could Sing:
A Look Into Hospice Music Therapy

By: Miranda Wall MT-BC

The Desk

Oh, hello there. You have found me. I am a desk. Not just any desk, though. I am the sturdy space where hospice stories begin. My surface hums with quiet purpose. I hold the echoes of tense care plan meetings, colleagues laughing over lunch, and holiday gatherings.

I can feel the faint grit of years settled into my surface, a mixture of pencil shavings, dust, and the occasional crumb from hurried lunches. The faint aroma of coffee clings to me, mingling with the sterile tang of hand sanitizer and the faint perfume of the people who sit here. Pens scratch across paper, keyboards click softly, and the hinge of the supervisor's chair lets out a low squeak that seems to punctuate the rhythm of the room. The hum of the overhead lights is constant, like a heartbeat I can feel beneath my polished veneer. Every sound, every smell, every texture is stored inside me, a library of subtle reminders that work, care, and life unfold here in measured, careful moments.

I notice the slight chill of the air conditioner brushing against my edges and the warmth that radiates from the sunlight spilling through the blinds, pooling in golden patches across my surface. The interview folder is smooth beneath a hand that trembles slightly, betraying the nerves it tries to hide. Paper rustles with each page turned, the faint whisper of ink scratching on sheets. Even the vibrations of the outside world creep in. The distant rumble of a passing truck, the faint chatter of staff in the hallway, the soft squeal of a rolling cart somewhere beyond the door. All of it dances over me, layers of the unseen, the unspoken, the almost imperceptible, creating a backdrop for the stories that will be written here, both on paper and in hearts.

Today, I am preparing for something new. A job interview. Not mine, of course. I am not the one seeking employment. But I will be the first to meet the music therapist who hopes to join this hospice team. The supervisor will sit next to me on her squeaky chair, a folder open and pen ready. The candidate will take the chair across, trying to calm her hands while explaining what it means to be a music therapist.

She will talk about the long road it took to get here. A bachelor's degree in music therapy. 1,200 hours of clinical training. Six months or more of an internship under supervision. A board certification exam. She will speak of their internship site, how she learned to listen for more than words, how she played to ease pain that medicine could not reach.

Later, I will witness the audition. The therapist will bring a guitar case that looks well-traveled, its handle worn smooth. Usually, another music therapist will join us, watching and listening to the one hoping to acquire this new position. They will jot something down. Probably about presence, tone, and how the therapist adjusts to spur of the moment requests.

The audition brings its own set of subtle notes. I feel the leather of the guitar case as it brushes my edge, the faint whiff of polished wood and worn fabric rising from it. Fingers pluck the strings with care, careful enough that each vibration seems to echo through me. I hear the soft intakes of breath, the almost imperceptible sighs as the candidate settles into a rhythm, and the scratching of pen across paper as the observing therapist notes something only they can catch. Even the way the chair legs scrape against the floor has a tone to it, a small punctuation that tells me when the energy in the room shifts. I feel it all, a tactile and auditory map of someone striving to be heard, to connect, to create.

By the time the paperwork begins, the room smells faintly of toner and the lingering floral of a hand lotion that someone applied in a rush. The weight of responsibility is tangible here, a quiet pressure that presses against me as I hold the folder and watch hand after hand sign, initial, and date. There is a rhythm to it, a ritual of preparation and consent, punctuated by the soft sighs of relief as boxes are checked and forms are completed. I feel the smooth, cold surface of each sheet, the indentation left by pens, and the subtle friction as pages shuffle together. So many papers. Background checks, health screenings, consent forms, confidentiality agreements. A small mountain of signatures before a single visit can happen. And by the end of the day, it will be quiet again. But I will feel the shift. The kind that happens when a new healer joins the rhythm of care.

And when the day winds down, the sounds fade. The sunlight shifts to softer, amber angles, the scent of coffee and ink lingers, and I am left quietly absorbing it all. I am a desk, yes, but I am also a witness. I feel every nervous pulse, every small victory, and every tiny moment that signals the beginning of someone new joining the rhythm of care. I have seen many professionals walk through the door, but there is something special about a music therapist. They do not just fill silence. They give it meaning. And soon, I will hear all the stories that follow.

The Trunk

Well, look who's here. It's very nice to meet you. I'm the trunk of this music therapist's car. Heavy, dependable, and don't you forget it. I've carried her gear through enough visits to fill a lifetime of stories, and I know her rhythm better than she knows her own heartbeat.

The smell hits first. A mixture of car leather warmed by the sun, faint traces of disinfectant from the wipes, and a lingering note of coffee from her travel mug that rests just beside me. The scent is familiar, comforting even, a signal that the day is about to begin. I feel the slight shift of the car as she eases her bag onto the seat, the faint vibration of the engine humming beneath me. Every tiny movement is magnified here. The snap of the seatbelt clicking, the soft rustle of paper from her notes, the gentle thump of the guitar case settling into place... These are the sounds that set the rhythm of our morning. Outside, tires hum along the pavement, muffled and distant. Inside, I am a stage, an anchor, and a silent witness to her preparation.

When the car stops, I sense the shift in energy before she even opens the door. The outside air carries a new set of smells: antiseptic from the building, faint flowers from the entryway, the subtle metallic tang of the elevator buttons she will press. The world beyond me is unpredictable. Voices drift in from hallways, shoes scuff against linoleum, doors click open and closed. Inside me, everything is calm. The instruments wait, ready and secure. I feel the unspoken trust she places in me, and I carry it like a weight I am proud to bear. Every note she will play, every rhythm she will coax from her patients, every smile and tear that crosses her path, it all begins here. And I am here too, solid, dependable, steady, quietly holding the center of it all.

With my door popped open, I notice that her hands are skilled, deliberate. I see the texture of the disinfectant wipes as they swipe over the guitar's wood, the tambourine's edges, the smooth shells of the egg shakers. Each wipe carries a soft swish and a faint chemical tang. She doesn't rush. She pauses, sometimes tilting an instrument just so, letting it catch the light, letting the surface breathe. Even after years of doing this, she treats each instrument with the same reverence she had the first day. I notice the subtle tension in her fingers, the tiny crease at her knuckles, the way she lifts her wrist to ensure every corner, every string, every hole is clean. It is a ritual, a meditation, a promise of safety and care. Not because anyone's watching. Not because she has to. She does it because it matters. Every time. Clean, ready, organized. No surprises. That's how you get the job done.

I see her checking her notes. Patient notes, preferences, mobility quirks. Even after years, she doesn't skim. She knows who startles, who prefers soft strumming, who can't handle a sudden beat. Experience talks, and she listens.

Back into me go the guitar, the tambourine, and the shakers. Stacked neatly. Every item in its place, no slipping, no banging around. She slams my lid shut, locks it down, and I swear you could hear a pin drop in here. Outside, the world is messy and unpredictable. Inside me, it's all business.

The interior of the car has its own quiet symphony. The gentle creak of the driver's seat as she adjusts, the soft click of her pen against the clipboard, the faint buzz of the air vents. The leather under me warms as the sun shifts, and I feel every bump in the road. Each instrument rests in its place, cushioned, secure, absorbing shocks and vibrations. I feel the weight of responsibility in these moments. The guitar, delicate and alive, trusts me to carry it safely. The tambourine waits quietly for its moment to shine, and the shakers sit snugly, ready to ripple rhythm into the air. I hold it all steady, a silent partner in this choreography of care, knowing that the smallest oversight could ripple through her session.

This music therapist sits quietly in the front seat and takes notes. I've watched her pick up the tiniest details, stuff you wouldn't even notice, and act like it's nothing. That's the sign of a pro. She doesn't make a fuss, she just does it. And when she steps out toward the building, instruments secure, wipes tucked away, I know every patient she meets will be safer for her having been there.

I've carried a lot in my years. But her guitar, tambourine, and shakers? They are in good hands. Every note she plays, every beat she shakes, it's all grounded in what I know she's learned the hard way: care is in the preparation, in the routine, in doing the small things right. And I'll be here to hold it all, like I always have.

The iPad

Hi there! I'm the iPad. I live in the music therapist's backpack, and I get to see everything that happens. Her whole job lives inside of me. I know it sounds a little boring, but it's really not! I get to hold all the important patient information, and I like keeping it safe and organized.

She opens me up, and I get to show her the list of patients for today. Names, notes, and everything else she could ever need. I love when she taps my screen and reads carefully. She notices things even I didn't expect her to notice. I hold all these little details for her so she can plan her sessions perfectly. She uses information from the nurses to make informed decisions during a new patient's evaluation.

I notice the small details that others might miss. The faint creak of a chair as someone shifts, the quiet sigh of a patient settling in, the shuffle of papers being pulled from a folder. I feel the cool glass beneath her fingers as she taps on me, each press a signal, a small command that she will act on it. I watch her adjust to what she finds, and sometimes I can sense the unspoken moments, the tiny decisions she makes to meet a patient where they are. I am part of the rhythm, even if it is subtle, even if no one else knows I am here.

She scrolls through me slowly sometimes, like she's reading a story. She checks for updates about her patients every day. I watch her think and plan. It's kind of like magic. I love being part of the magic. I beep softly to remind her if something is missing on a form, and she smiles at me and fixes it right away.

There are times when she pauses to think. I feel the weight of her hand resting on me as she reviews her notes, her thumb brushing over the edge, lingering. The faint scent of coffee or hand sanitizer drifts in the air. Outside, sunlight shifts across the room, casting slanted shadows on the floor. Inside, I hum quietly with the energy of anticipation, of planning, of care. I am always alert, ready to hold the next observation, the next insight, the next detail she will need to guide her session with precision and compassion.

I also notice her moments of exhaustion. The long days, the countless rooms, the repetitions of the same motions can tire her. Her voice grows hoarse, her hands linger a fraction longer on a page, her eyes blink more frequently. I am there to help her pause, to give her space to recalibrate, to remind her of the details she has captured so she does not have to carry it all in her memory alone. The smoothness of my screen and the gentle hum when I alert her are small comforts, subtle tools that keep her present, keep her able to do the work she loves so deeply.

I can tell she's been doing this a long time. Even though I'm just a tablet, I can feel her confidence. She knows how to keep people safe, how to pick the right music, and how to make every moment meaningful. I don't get to play the songs myself, but I get to help her make sure every note is just right.

When she's done with me, she tucks me back in her backpack, safe and clean, ready for the next visit. I get to rest for a little while, but I know I'll be needed again soon. When the day ends, and she tucks me back into the backpack, I feel the shift from activity to rest. The world outside moves on in a blur of tires, footsteps, and wind. Inside me, the patient histories, the schedules, the observations, the reminders, all settle quietly. I hold them for her, steady, protected, waiting for the next time she opens me, the next room she enters, the next moment she will create with music and care. I am small and silent, but I carry a weight that is essential, and that weight makes me proud. I love that she trusts me to hold all the important information. I like helping her make music that makes people feel better. Even if I'm just a little screen with buttons, I get to be part of something really big. And that makes me happy.

The Guitar Case

Hey. I'm the guitar case. I've been around long enough to know my role. I get carried into countless rooms, holding both comfort and grief, and then I get set down. Across the room, out of the way. Not touched again until it's time to leave. That's fine with me. I don't need attention. I just need to be ready.

She unzips me gently, pulls out the guitar. Sometimes she reaches back into me for a capo or an extra pick. I hand them over without complaint. I don't mind waiting. Patience is part of my job.

Sometimes I catch the faint scent of disinfectant from her wipes, mixed with the warm wood of the guitar that still lingers inside me. It is a blend that never quite fades, even after years. When she lifts the guitar out, I feel the cool air rush in, brushing over the soft interior lining that cradles the shape of the instrument. The zipper glides open with a quiet rasp, familiar and steady, followed by the faint creak of the strap as she adjusts it over her shoulder. These are small sounds, ordinary to anyone else, but to me, they are the rhythm of purpose.

I also have a bigger job no one really thinks about. I protect the most important instrument during travel, through the car, down elevators, down hallways, through doorways. Every bump, every jostle, every tilt of the cart or lift, I absorb it all. The guitar is delicate, and I make sure it arrives safe, steady, and ready. That is why I am built strong and padded. I take that responsibility seriously.

She starts with the patient. I sit across the room, watching and feeling the vibrations of each note, absorbing the quiet moments. The soft hums, the tiny smiles, the moments that don't need words. She adjusts her approach as she goes, notices small cues, records her observations in her notebook or iPad. I stay put, calm, ready, but out of the way. I like it this way. I like knowing I'm trusted, that she knows how to use me, and that I'll be ready when she needs me again.

When we enter a patient's room, I am set down gently, always in a corner or by the window. From here, I watch it all. The scent of lotion and the faint trace of coffee drift through the air. Machines hum softly, rhythmic and steady. Sometimes a curtain sways with the smallest movement of air from the vent above. There is a tenderness in the quiet. I can feel the vibration of her guitar through the floor, low and steady, like a heartbeat beneath everything else. It reaches me, even from across the room.

I listen to the music fill the space, the strumming calm and patient. Each note seems to linger longer in rooms like these. There are times when I sense something shift. The tone of her voice softens, or a patient's breathing slows, or someone nearby exhales, the sound weighted with both relief and grief. The world outside this room fades. Only the music remains. I stay still, taking it all in. I do not need to play or move. My role is simple but important. I am the quiet constant, the one that holds what matters when the sound fades away.

When the session ends, she wipes down the strings, the fretboard, her hands. I smell the faint citrus of her disinfectant again, mixed with the clean air from the open door. The guitar rests back inside me, warm from her touch, and I close around it carefully. The zipper slides shut, sealing in the echoes of the room we just left. Outside, the hallway hums with footsteps and soft voices. Inside me, it is still. I like it that way. I keep the guitar safe until the next song begins. Notes recorded, instruments cleaned, everything in order. I rest until the next visit, quiet and content. I don't need to be the star. I just need to be ready, steady, and calm. That is enough. That is always enough. That is my job. That is my peace.

The Window

Hello. I am the window. I watch everything that happens in this room. I see sunlight spill across the floor, shadows stretch and shrink, and the seasons change outside my glass. I have seen quiet mornings, soft afternoons, and evenings filled with whispers.

The air in the room always carries a certain texture. In the morning, it smells faintly of coffee and freshly folded linens. By afternoon, there might be a trace of floral lotion or the faint metallic scent from medical equipment. When visitors arrive, the air shifts again, touched with perfume, outdoor chill, or the sweet scent of bakery goods tucked into paper bags. I breathe it all in through the smallest cracks along my frame, collecting the sensory fingerprints of every story that passes through this space.

Outside, the world never stops. Birds perch on the sill, chirping in brief bursts before they flit away. Trees sway and whisper secrets to each other, their leaves brushing softly against the glass when the wind picks up. I listen to rain when it comes, tapping gently at first, then steady and rhythmic, a quiet duet with the music inside. Snow muffles the world, dimming every sound, until the only thing that seems to exist is the strum of a guitar and the sound of someone's soft breathing nearby.

Sometimes the room is full of laughter. A patient taps along with the guitar, a tiny smile spreading across their face. Sometimes there are tears, and the music seems to hold them gently, like a hand resting on a shoulder. I have seen families gather, holding hands, leaning in close, sharing memories and stories in hushed voices. I have seen moments of surprise, when a patient remembers a song from long ago, eyes lighting up as if no time has passed at all.

Sometimes the room is still. Silence settles like a soft blanket. The guitar rests across the therapist's lap, and even the smallest hum carries weight. I watch as people breathe, as they look at each other, as they simply exist together in these quiet moments. I have seen conversations start and stop, tears come and go, and small victories unfold without a sound.

I have seen anger, frustration, and confusion pass across faces. I have seen fear ease with the first gentle strum of the guitar. I have seen hope rekindle, sadness soften, and peace arrive, sometimes in a single note.

I have learned that every day looks the same to me, yet feels entirely different. Some sessions begin with energy, the guitar bright and quick, sunlight dancing across the room. Other days are quieter, heavier, as if the very air is holding its breath. I watch the therapist read the room like a musician reads a score, adjusting tempo and tone without a word. I see her eyes flicker with understanding, her body moving in rhythm with the emotion that fills the space. It is something beyond training. It is instinct, care, and connection blended into one seamless motion.

When evening arrives, I hold the fading light as long as I can. The golden glow spills across the bed, touches the guitar's surface, and paints the walls in soft amber. Then the color fades, and the music slows, until the final note hovers and disappears into the quiet. I watch her gather her things, her shoulders both heavy and at peace. The room falls still again, and I reflect the last bit of light until it fades completely. Night settles, and I wait. The next day will bring a new melody, a new story, another small moment that I will quietly hold. I wait for the next person to enter, for the next song to be played, for the next story to unfold. I see it all, every day, and I hold it quietly, like a witness to life's small miracles.

The Hallway

I'm the hallway. Long, narrow, and endlessly patient. I see everything, and I mean everything. The way her shoes click against my floor, the soft shuffle of a visitor's slippers, the quiet sigh of someone lost in thought. I know the rhythm of this place better than anyone, but don't get me wrong... I don't get bored. There's always something to notice.

She walks my length a lot. Sometimes she's in a hurry, like she's racing the clock, and sometimes she drifts, leaning into a quiet moment with a patient. She trusts me to hold her steps, to give her space, and I do. I've learned that routines are important, but rigidity is for someone else. She bends, she adjusts, she improvises, and I roll with it.

Doors open, doors close, laughter floats down from a room, a murmur drifts my way. I catch the tiny details most people miss. A patient hesitates before letting go of a hand. A staff member lingers a beat too long, thinking about what they just said. She notices these things too, but she moves fast enough to keep the flow.

I've seen routines repeat for years and yet never be exactly the same. That's the beauty of this place. Flexibility is built into every step, every session, every hallway crossing. And I? I carry it all. Quiet, steady, a little knowing, a little sarcastic if you read between the lines, but always ready for the next footstep, the next bend, the next change in rhythm.

When the air conditioner hums, I feel the faint vibration ripple through me like a pulse. The scent of disinfectant mixes with hints of lavender from someone's lotion, a strange kind of balance between sterile and soft. Sometimes, a tray of coffee rolls by, steam rising in little ghosts that fade before reaching my ceiling. Other times, I smell the faint sweetness of flowers delivered to a room, bright against the usual stillness. I absorb it all, let it echo through my length like memory, sharp, fleeting, and real.

At night, I quiet down. The lights dim, and my floor grows cool, the shine of daytime footsteps softening into shadow. I listen to the faint whir of machines behind closed doors, the creak of old pipes settling in. Once in a while, she walks me even then, her steps slower, more thoughtful, maybe heavier. The air feels different, thicker somehow. I keep her company, guiding her from room to room, no words needed.

Sometimes, I think I carry emotion the way she carries music. Grief, hope, exhaustion, they all trail behind her and sink into my walls. I've learned the difference between the shuffle of sorrow and the stride of relief. I've learned how silence can feel full, and how laughter can echo long after everyone's gone. I hold it all, quietly, never asking to let go.

I stretch on, patient and watchful, keeping track of patterns, pauses, and the odd little surprises that make this place live. I am the hallway. I see it all. I hear it all. And I am always here, ready for the next step.

The Blanket

Hello, dear. I'm the blanket. Soft, warm, and always here. I wrap around shoulders, curl around laps, and sometimes rest lightly over arms. I feel every sigh, every tremble, every shiver. And when the music begins, I notice the little miracles that happen without anyone asking.

A strum of the guitar, a gentle note in the air, and the body responds on its own. A finger taps a rhythm, a foot sways, a head nods, a breath catches. These are the invisible dances of the brain, tiny connections forming and sparking without thought. Music wakes memories, stirs emotions, nudges the body, and the mind follows.

I've felt hands that barely move squeeze in time with a beat. I've felt toes curl, smiles appear, eyes brighten, all before a word is spoken. Music finds the pathways, the neurons that remember, that connect sound to feeling and motion. And I wrap around it all, quietly holding, softly comforting, letting the warmth settle in with every note.

Sometimes the responses are gentle, subtle, and almost shy. Sometimes they surprise, bringing laughter, tears, or memories long tucked away. Every chord, every hum, every strum is a bridge, and I am here to hold it, to hold them, to make them feel safe as their bodies and hearts respond.

When the session ends, I fold softly, carrying the warmth and the echoes of music in my fibers. The moments remain, tucked gently in the mind and the heart, and I stay here, comforting, nurturing, quietly proud of every connection made, every little response sparked.

And oh, the textures of this place. I feel the rough edges of wheelchairs brush against me, the smoothness of a patient's skin beneath my folds, the faint scent of lotion and antiseptic mingling in the air. Sometimes, a bit of sunlight slips through the blinds and settles on me, warming the fabric like a soft breath. Other times, it's the chill of the air vent that reminds me to cling tighter, to lend my warmth to whoever needs it most.

The room hums with gentle sounds. The low murmur of voices, the soft strum of guitar strings, the whisper of shoes on linoleum. I absorb every vibration, every flicker of sound that ripples through the air. I can almost feel the rhythm pulsing beneath my fibers, like a heartbeat shared between the therapist and the patient. It moves through me, steady and kind.

I've learned that touch carries its own kind of language. A nurse's gentle adjustment of my edges, a family member smoothing me across a loved one's legs, the therapist tucking me closer when a shiver passes. Each touch holds care, gratitude, sometimes even goodbye. I keep these gestures stored within me like quiet prayers, never forgotten.

And when night comes, when the guitar case is closed and the hallway stills, I rest draped over the arm of a chair. I remember the laughter, the tremors of memory, the soft songs that stirred the air. I may be just a blanket, but I have held moments too fragile for words. I have been witness to comfort, to healing, to grace that slips in between notes. I will be ready again tomorrow, waiting to wrap the next story in warmth.

The Wristwatch

Hello. I'm the wristwatch. I sit here, snug against her wrist, quietly keeping track of everything. The seconds tick by, the minutes pass, and I watch it all unfold. Some visits feel fast, full of energy and movement. Other visits feel slow, heavy with emotion, or soft with quiet reflection. Time keeps ticking, steady and unchanging, but each visit is different, and I feel it all.

I notice the rhythms. She strums the guitar, and her hands move in time, sometimes slow, sometimes fast, always following the pulse of the room. I mark the pauses, the brief hesitations, the gentle adjustments. I know when she leans in to listen, when she waits, when she guides, and when she steps back. Time matters, but she does not let it control her. Flexibility is her rhythm, and I follow along.

I see beginnings and endings. She checks her notes, glances at me, adjusts a string, strums one last chord. The session wraps up. I witness every routine, the setup, the playing, the recording, the cleanup, and yet each day is never the same. I keep track, quietly, noticing how the same minute can feel full of discovery or heavy with pause.

Some moments are fleeting. A smile, a breath caught in recognition, a hand tapping lightly to a beat. I notice them all. I count the seconds, but I also feel the spaces between them, the silence, the pause, the gentle stretch of time where the unexpected happens.

When the session ends, she sets me down, checks the next appointment, and moves forward. I keep ticking. Always counting, always aware, always ready to mark another moment, another rhythm, another life touched by music.

But I also feel the weight of it. The tired pulse beneath my band, the faint tremor in her wrist when the day runs long. I sense her exhaustion, though she hides it well. Sometimes, when she exhales between sessions, I can almost hear her heart slowing down, gathering itself before the next doorway opens. It's in those seconds that I understand what it means to carry the stories of others.

I've heard laughter echo through the hall, the sharp cry of a monitor, the quiet sigh of relief when a patient's eyes flutter closed. Each sound becomes a measure of time for me. I tick through it all, unblinking, but not untouched. Even the silence between songs feels heavy, almost sacred, as if the air itself is holding its breath.

When sunlight hits my face just right, I catch the glint of her pulse beneath me. It's steady, even when her day is not. I think about all the seconds I've counted and how many of them have held something more than time. They've held connection, courage, endings, and beginnings. She trusts me to keep her grounded, to keep her aware of when to begin and when to let go.

And when the night finally comes, and she slips me off her wrist, I rest in quiet gratitude. My hands still move, my gears still hum, but my purpose feels different. I have measured not just hours, but moments that will never repeat. Tomorrow, I'll do it again. Quietly, faithfully, always in rhythm with the heart that wears me.

The Guitar

It's me, hi, I'm the guitar. Some call me the star of the show. I get carried to every visit and what can I say? I'm the attention grabber. People will stop us in the hallway to ask, "Is that a guitar?" Yes, hello! It's me. But don't think I'm the cool one. I get strummed, tuned, and occasionally talked to. But I'm not just a prop. I see the work she puts in, and let me tell you, it is a lot.

When we get home, she logs onto her computer like a tiny research factory. Articles, courses, videos, she absorbs it all. And then she comes to me. Fingers pressing, strumming, plucking, over and over, trying that new chord or tricky pattern. Honestly, I have lost count of how many times she has done the same chord. I have blisters myself from thinking about it. But she does not stop until it is perfect. And I know why. She wants her patients to have the best, no compromises.

I have seen her grow over the years. I have seen her adapt songs, improvise, figure out ways to reach someone who does not respond at first. I have been in rooms where laughter erupted from a single strum and in rooms where silence held everything. She learns from all of it and I get the privilege of feeling it all firsthand.

And yes, sometimes I get tossed aside while she experiments, muttering, testing, tweaking. Fine. I do not mind. I have patience and I know the moment she nails it, I will be the one to carry that perfection into the next room.

I travel with her every day, through hallways, doors, and rooms. I see her dedication in action and in practice. I hear her determination in every note she plays. I might be a little worn around the edges, but I have stories, and I know quality when I see it. She is constantly growing, constantly learning, and I get a front-row seat. And that is a pretty good view if you ask me.

But let me tell you something most people do not notice. When she practices late into the evening, the house gets quiet. The world outside hums with night sounds, and it is just her and me. The air smells faintly of coffee and lemon-scented cleaner. Her fingertips are red, calloused, and steady. She hums softly under her breath, and I feel her heartbeat through the vibration of my strings. This is where growth happens. Quietly. Patiently. Without applause.

There are moments when she stops playing and just listens. The faint buzz of a fluorescent light, the creak of the chair beneath her, the way her breath slows before she starts again. Those pauses matter as much as the music. They teach her presence, patience, timing. I like to think I help her with that. Every strum that lands just right, every chord that resonates deeper than before, it's because we've learned how to listen together.

And when the morning light filters in through the blinds, she picks me up again. The scent of coffee returns, warm and familiar. She runs her thumb across my neck, checking the tuning, adjusting a string that slipped overnight. She's not just a therapist. She's a student, a scholar, an artist always reaching for better. I get to witness it all.

By the time we leave for work, the world is still waking up. She carries me with purpose, her steps measured and sure. I rest against her side, feeling the rhythm of her walk and the hum of her breath. We've got another day ahead of us. Another chance to make something meaningful. And as always, I'll be ready.

The Hospital Bed

Hello. I am the hospital bed. I hold them all. I feel their weight, their weakness, their quiet breaths. I have seen sorrow and relief, the small smiles that hide great sadness, the tears that fall silently. I have held bodies that will leave me soon, and I have held those who linger a little longer, and in both, I feel the heaviness of it all.

She comes to me every day. She watches, she listens, she notes. Fingers tap lightly on her iPad, recording the responses, the progress, the small victories. Sometimes the patient moves, sometimes they do not. Sometimes their eyes brighten with recognition, sometimes they close in quiet resignation. She notices it all, every twitch, every sigh, every pause, and she writes it down. The work is never easy. The endings are never easy.

When it is time to finish, she does it with care. She eases them, reassures them, sings the last note, strums the last chord, lets the music fade gently into the quiet of the room. I feel the tension leave their bodies, but I also feel the weight of what lingers. Some departures are just for the day, some feel like the last. She knows the difference, but even she cannot take away the grief.

I have seen her close sessions softly, quietly, always aware of safety, always aware of comfort, always aware of the fragility of life. I feel the endings as deeply as she does. I see the notes recorded, the reflections made, the plans for tomorrow. But I also feel the emptiness when the room is empty, the echo of voices that will not return, the stillness that follows.

I hold them all. The laughter, the grief, the hope, the quiet resignation. I am steady beneath them, but I am heavy with what I witness. Each session ends, each life moves forward, and I am left with the memory of both joy and sorrow. I am the hospital bed. I hold, I remember, and I grieve with them all.

Sometimes I feel the music through the mattress before I hear it. The vibration moves through me, faint and steady, like a heartbeat. It reaches the patient first, then settles into the room. I can tell when the notes are meant for comfort, for courage, or for farewell. Each sound has its own weight. Some feel light as air, some press into me, sinking deep into the folds of the blanket. I hold it all, even the echoes that linger after she leaves.

I have learned the rhythm of this work. The quiet greetings, the adjustments of pillows, the careful touch of her hand on a wrist or shoulder. She always checks that the patient is safe, comfortable, seen. The music is not just played, it is offered. A gift, a bridge, a way to say what words cannot. I am the stage for those unspoken exchanges, the place where love and loss meet without needing explanation.

When the room grows still again, I hear her exhale softly. She gathers her things with care, never in a rush. I can feel the sadness she carries, but also the gratitude. She has given something of herself, and she leaves a piece of comfort behind. I feel it too, that quiet balance of letting go and holding on.

The room grows dim as the day ends. The hum of machines softens, the air grows heavy, and I wait for the next arrival. I never know if it will be a beginning or an ending, but I am ready. I am built to hold, to comfort, to bear the weight of everything that passes through. And in the quiet that follows each song, I stay. Listening. Remembering. Always here.

The Water Bottle

Oh, hello! I am the water bottle. I ride in her bag, rest in the car's cupholder, and sit beside her chair. I am always within reach, a small but crucial part of her day. My surface often feels cool to her touch in the morning, fresh from the sink or the fridge. Condensation slides down my sides, leaving little rings of moisture wherever I go. She sometimes forgets me, caught up in her rhythm of care, her guitar, her notes. But I am here to remind her that she matters too.

Her days are long. I travel with her through quiet halls, patient rooms, and warm car rides between visits. I hear her voice rise and fall, sometimes bright and clear, sometimes soft and tired. By afternoon, her throat begins to ache, her words come slower, and that is when she reaches for me. The first sip always seems to wake her up a little, the sound of the cap twisting open, the faint squeak as I bend, the cool rush that washes over her dry throat. She exhales, steadier, calmer, and goes back to the work that fills her heart even when it drains her body.

I have seen her pause mid-song, hand brushing against me as if in silent gratitude. Sometimes the air in the room feels heavy, thick with emotion, and I can almost sense her heartbeat quicken. She takes a sip, lets the water sit in her mouth before swallowing, as though grounding herself. Those moments are small but powerful. They remind her that she is human too, warm, breathing, tired, alive.

She cares for others endlessly, but she is learning to care for herself too. Before each session, she fills me halfway with cold water, knowing it will be just right after an hour of singing. She rinses me at night, scrubbing away the faint scent of coffee from earlier in the day. The sound of running water, the clink of metal against the sink, it all becomes part of her nightly ritual, quiet and grounding. I wait, clean and ready for tomorrow, like she tries to be.

There are days she forgets me entirely. I sit untouched in the car, feeling the warmth build as the sun creeps across the dashboard. She returns hours later, voice rough, shoulders heavy, and I know she pushed herself too far again. When she finally drinks, she closes her eyes for a second longer than usual, as if the water could wash away the exhaustion itself.

I witness her small routines, the way she twists my lid open during charting, how she takes a sip before pulling out of the parking lot, how she tucks me beside her guitar case before heading inside. I see how each gulp restores her, how it steadies her breathing and her mind. Without that care, her music, her warmth, her compassion, all of it would begin to fade.

I am small, quiet, ordinary. But in this life of music, care, and constant motion, I am essential. I remind her that she cannot pour from an empty cup. I support her so she can support others. And when she finally sits at home at the end of the day, hand resting on my side, I feel the gentle rhythm of her gratitude, unspoken but full of life.

The Egg Shakers

Ch ch. Ch ch. We are the egg shakers. Small, unassuming, but we have a job. We travel in a bag, bouncing lightly with her steps, feeling the gentle sway as she walks down hallways, and we wait patiently for the moment we are needed. The leather of our bag is smooth and worn, the faint scent of disinfectant and faint coffee clinging to it. Today, that moment comes in the memory care room.

The room is filled with voices, some clear, some lost in the fog of forgetting. Sunlight filters through the blinds, casting stripes across the floor, warm and soft. She greets them all, her smile steady, her eyes attentive, and we are lifted, one in each hand. Suddenly the room has a pulse. We rattle in time with her guidance, tiny beads inside us colliding gently, a soft, soothing sound that draws hands together, coax smiles, spark recognition.

Some follow immediately, shaking us in rhythm, their hands warm and uncertain at first. Others hesitate, fingers brushing lightly against our smooth shells, movements slow, cautious. That is fine. She adjusts, counting softly, offering encouragement in her voice, showing the motion herself. We feel the small victories: fingers tapping in unison, heads nodding to the beat, a laugh breaking through a long silence, the faint creak of chairs as participants sway.

We know the patterns she uses, the songs that often bring memories back, the ones that linger longer in the air. We sense her energy, the slight tension in her shoulders as she anticipates who will join in, the tiny shifts of her hands guiding us. She watches closely, notes subtle cues, smiles at progress, and never rushes anyone. The session flows, sometimes fast, sometimes slow, always careful, always patient.

The air smells faintly of sanitizer, a soft mix of cleaning supplies and the faint sweetness of lotions, mingling with the warm hum of conversation. When the song ends, we are set aside again, still vibrating with the echo of their energy. We see the tiny connections formed, the joy in recognition, and the gentle reassurance she gives when someone struggles.

By the end of the session, she collects us, shakes off our dust, and places us carefully back in our bag. The fabric is slightly rough against our shells, a comforting texture after a session of motion. We rest, but we remember. We remember the laughter, the hesitation, the small triumphs, the tiny sparks of memory that light up the room. Every tap, every shake, every smile is etched into us. We are small, but our purpose is mighty: to bring rhythm, connection, and life to moments that need it most.

Sometimes we can still feel the warmth of hands lingering, the faint echoes of the last note reverberating against our bodies. We rest quietly, ready for the next room, the next song, the next opportunity to help memories surface, smiles bloom, and hearts connect. We are egg shakers, small but essential, carrying not just rhythm, but fragments of joy, courage, and remembrance wherever we go.

The Last Breath

I am the last breath. I come quietly, almost unseen, yet heavy with all that has passed. I carry the tremors of laughter, the faint echoes of song, the warmth of hands that have held and been held. The air tastes faintly of antiseptic and lavender, mingling with the lingering scent of worn blankets and polished wood. I am soft, fleeting, yet charged with weight. I am watched. I am feared. I am inevitable.

I drift through the room as her music floats, each note a gentle tide. The vibrations of the guitar ripple through the floor, through the blankets, through the still bodies resting beneath. I feel the subtle warmth of skin against fabric, the coolness of air moving across pillows, the faint tremor of a hand trying to tap a rhythm one last time. The sound of her voice is a thread in the quiet, tremulous but steady, carrying reassurance that even I, the final exhale, am not alone.

I linger in the pauses, in the moments between strums, where the room holds its breath. The soft rustle of sheets, the distant hum of the air purifier, the gentle creak of the bed frame as it shifts slightly, all of it marks my presence. I hover around the smallest details, the flutter of an eyelid, the shallow inhale that marks the nearing of release, the subtle pulse of a heartbeat slowing beneath a chest that has borne much. I am heavy, yet I float, delicate yet insistent.

The room is alive with invisible currents. I feel the lingering heat of sunlight from the window, brushing against walls, pooling on the floor in golden rectangles. A clock ticks somewhere, a metronome for the fragile rhythm of life that remains. I taste the cool metallic tang of the oxygen mask, smell the faint perfume of someone who once visited, and hear the soft creak of shoes stepping lightly outside the door. Each sensory note wraps around me as I prepare for what must come.

She plays on, but I can see her awareness of my approach. The strings vibrate differently now, softer, slower, more deliberate. The vibrations ripple through her fingertips into the air and into me. I feel the subtle quiver in the blankets, the faint rise and fall of a chest, the delicate press of a hand on a wrist to reassure that release is gentle. The music curves around me, cradles me, and guides me like a river bending into the last quiet bay.

I am the hush after the final note, the weight of all that has been lived, the silence that carries memory. I feel the warmth of a hand linger on a shoulder, the faint smell of disinfectant giving way to the scent of home in the room. I sense the tension leaving the space, leaving bodies, leaving hearts. I am both the end and the bridge, the moment of calamity softened by care. I leave traces in the vibrating air, in the faint echo of song, in the invisible threads connecting those who remain to what has passed.

I am the last breath. I am feared because I end, yet I am sacred because I release. I carry sorrow and peace in equal measure, the weight of endings and the shimmer of what remains. I leave the room altered, quiet, charged with remembrance. The song lingers, the touch lingers, and in that, I persist beyond myself.

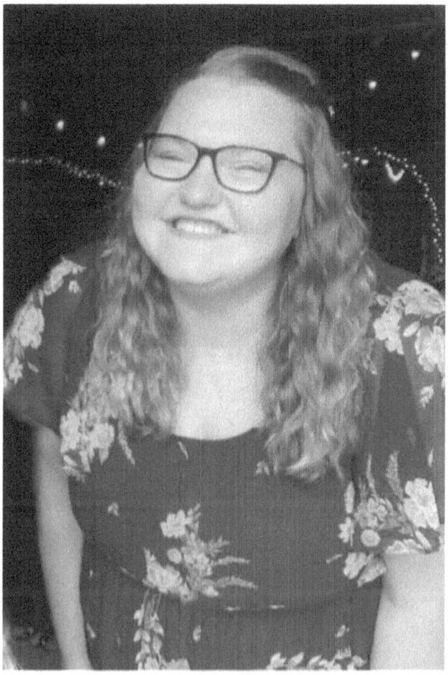

About the Author

Miranda Wall, MT-BC, is a board-certified music therapist with a passion for bringing comfort, connection, and dignity to individuals in hospice and end-of-life care. Through her clinical work, she has witnessed the profound ways music can ease pain, spark memories, and create moments of presence when words are not enough. In *If Things Could Sing*, Miranda blends her experience and creativity to illuminate the quiet, transformative power of music therapy, giving voice to the unseen work that heals hearts and honors life's final chapters.

www.ingramcontent.com/pod-product-compliance
Lightning Source LLC
LaVergne TN
LVHW090433210926
848480LV00002B/816